Ashwagandha

The Miraculous Herb!
Holistic Solutions & Proven Healing Recipes for Health, Beauty, Weight Loss & Hormone Balance

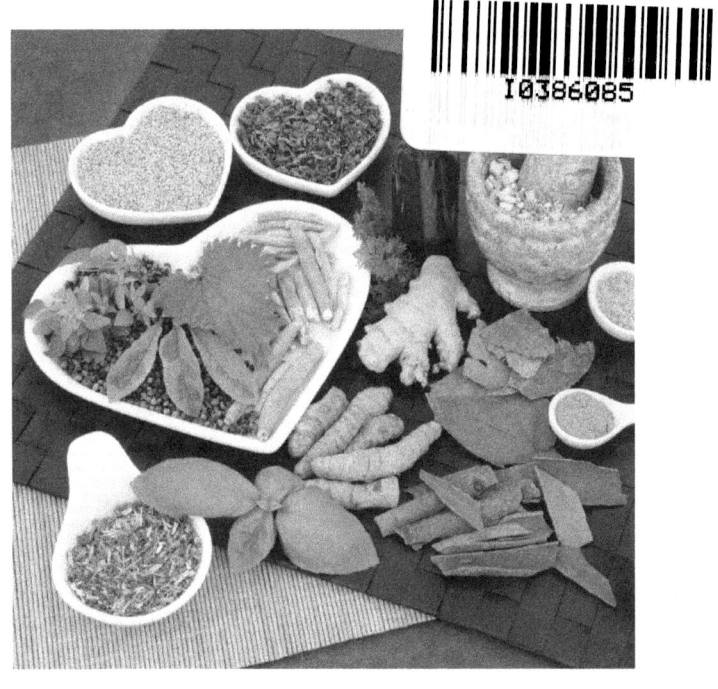

by Elena Garcia

Copyright Elena Garcia © 2016

www.YourWellnessBooks.com

All rights reserved. No part of this publication may be reproduced, stored in a retrieval system, or transmitted, in any form or by any means, electronic, mechanical, photocopying, recording or otherwise, without the prior written permission of the author and the publishers.

The scanning, uploading, and distribution of this book via the Internet or via any other means without the permission of the author is illegal and punishable by law. Please purchase only authorized electronic editions, and do not participate in or encourage electronic piracy of copyrighted materials.

Legal Notice:

This book is copyright protected. It for personal use only. You cannot amend, distribute, sell, use, quote or paraphrase any part or the content within this book without the consent of the author or copyright owner. Legal action will be pursued if this is breached.

Disclaimer Notice:

Please note the information contained within this document is for educational and entertainment purposes only. Every attempt has been made to provide accurate, up to date and completely reliable information. No warranties of any kind are expressed or implied.

Readers acknowledge that the author is not engaging in the rendering of legal, financial, medical or professional advice. By reading this document, the reader agrees that under no circumstances are we responsible for any losses, direct or indirect, which are incurred as a result of the use of information contained within this document, including, but not limited to, errors, omissions, or inaccuracies.

Contents

Ashwagandha: Introduction...5

Chapter 1...15

The Astonishing Uses and Benefits of Ashwagandha

Chapter 2...33

How to Use it Safely & Wisely: Side-Effects and Precautions of Using Ashwagandha

Chapter 3...38

Mouth-Watering Smoothie Recipes using Ashwagandha

In Conclusion...69

Ashwagandha: Introduction

Ashwagandha is also known as Indian ginseng and is widely used within Ayurvedic healing practices. Ayurveda is an ancient holistic healing practice that originated in the Indian subcontinent. This legendary healing practice began with tales of how the Gods would empower the sages with knowledge around this healing practice that the sages would then pass on to human physicians of the time. As with many ancient healing practices Ayurvedic healing has developed and evolved over the course of the last two millennia into what we know it to be today; however it is still largely based on the ancient traditions and methods.

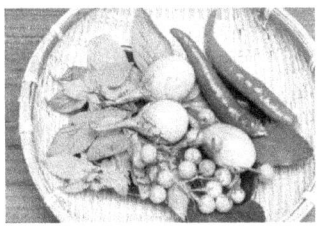

Some Background on Ayurveda:

The theories and practices of Ayurveda are largely based on the use of ancient yet complex herbal compounds, and the evolution of the practice began to introduce the use of mineral compounds within the healing processes as well. The ancient practices of Ayurveda also taught surgical techniques such as rhinoplasty (which is essentially a nose job), basic suturing or the stitching of wounds, and the extraction of foreign objects.

The basis of Ayurvedic practice works on three elemental substances known as *doshas*, these doshas are referred to as *Pitta, Vata and Kapha*, and the belief is that if these doshas are balanced then the body is in a healthy state, but if these doshas are out of balance then the body is in a state of dis-ease and therefore will be needing treatment.

Ayurvedic practice consists of eight accepted components which were derived from ancient Sanskrit literature. These eight components include the practices of the following:

- General medicine and medicine of the body
- The treatment of children (pediatrics)
- Surgical techniques and the extraction of foreign objects
- The treatment of ailments affecting the ears, eyes, nose and mouth (what we know as ENT or ear, nose and throat treatment)
- The pacification of possessing spirits and the extracting of these sprits from those whom they are possessing.
- Toxicology

- Rejuvenation and tonics for increasing lifespan, intellect and strength

- Aphrodisiacs and fertility treatments

When looking at the principles of Ayurveda one will notice that an emphasis is put on the obtaining and maintaining of balance within the body, mind and spirit in order to achieve a holistic state of health and wellness. The practice of Ayurveda cautions people to stay within the limits of reasonable balance and to maintain self awareness when following nature's urges; therefore one is encouraged to moderate food intake, sleep and sexual intercourse.

Doctors specializing and practicing Ayurveda regard the physical existence, mental existence and personality as unit, with each of these components having the ability to influence each other. This approach is taken when diagnosing and treating a patient's ailments. There is another part of Ayurveda that states that the body has channels which transport fluids and that these channels can be opened up and treated through massage therapy using oils. Unhealthy or blocked channels are thought to cause diseases.

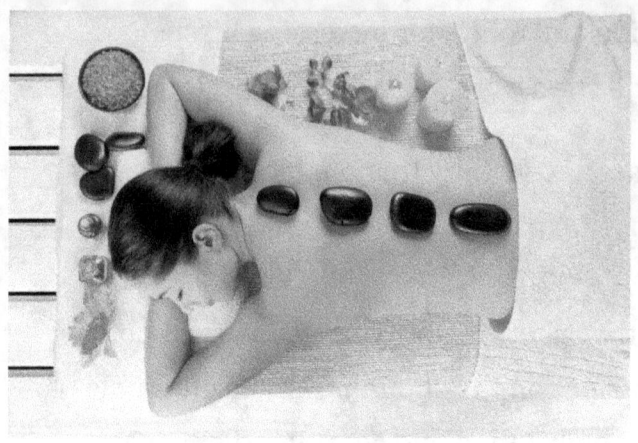

Ayurveda uses eight approaches in order to diagnose illnesses, these approaches include:

- Pulse

- Urine

- Stool

- Tongue

- Speech

- Touch

- Vision

- Appearance

The five senses are always used when approaching diagnosis.

Ayurveda places an emphasis on obtaining and maintaining vitality by building a healthy metabolic system, which consistently possesses a healthy state of digestion and excretion. Ayurveda also places a focus on exercise such as the practice of yoga and meditation. There is also a focus on the maintenance of natural cycles of sleep, waking, working and meditation in order to achieve a state of good health. Personal hygiene, including regular bathing, cleaning of teeth and hair, skin and eye washing are also central to obtaining and maintaining a state of good health.

Ayurvedic treatments include the use of substances that are derived from roots, fruits, seeds, bark and leaves. There are some instances where treatments will call for the use of mineral substances such as sulfur, copper sulfate, lead and gold. Ayurveda will also sometimes use alcoholic beverages as forms of treatment. However many of the most common and well known Ayurvedic treatments are based on the use of herbal remedies.

More about Ashwangandha:

When it comes to the healing practices of Ayurveda, Ashwagandha is considered one the most powerful herbs. The name of the herb comes from the Sanskrit texts and when translated into English means *"the smell of a horse"*, which indicates that it imparts the strength and vigor of a strong stallion. Ashwagandha has been traditionally prescribed to help people recover and strengthen their immune systems after suffering from an illness.

Ashwagandha, although referred to as *"Indian Ginseng"*, due to its rejuvenating properties, it actually has no botanical connection to ginseng at all. Ashwagandha is actually part of the tomato family and is a small, plump shrub that has oval leaves and yellow flowers; the fruit that it bears is about the size of a raisin. This herb is native to growing in the dry regions of India, North Africa, the Middle East and more recently some areas of the United States.

Ashwagandha is known as an adaptogenic herb. Adaptogens are substances such as amino acids, vitamins and herbs that modulate the body's response to stress and/or a changing environment, both of which are consistent aspect of modern day life. Adaptogens are known to help the body cope with and fight against external stressors such as toxins and the environment, as well as internal stressors such as anxiety, insomnia and depression.

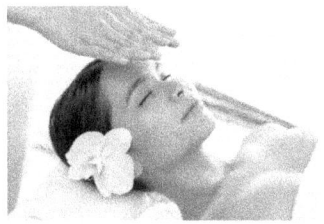

Ashwagandha has many useful medicinal chemical properties such as withanolides, (which are steroidal lactones), alkaloids, choline, fatty acids, amino acids and a variety of naturally occurring sugars. The leaves and the fruit of the Ashwagandha plant possess very valuable therapeutic and healing properties; however it is the root of the plant that is most commonly used in the more Western practices of Ayurveda and its treatments.

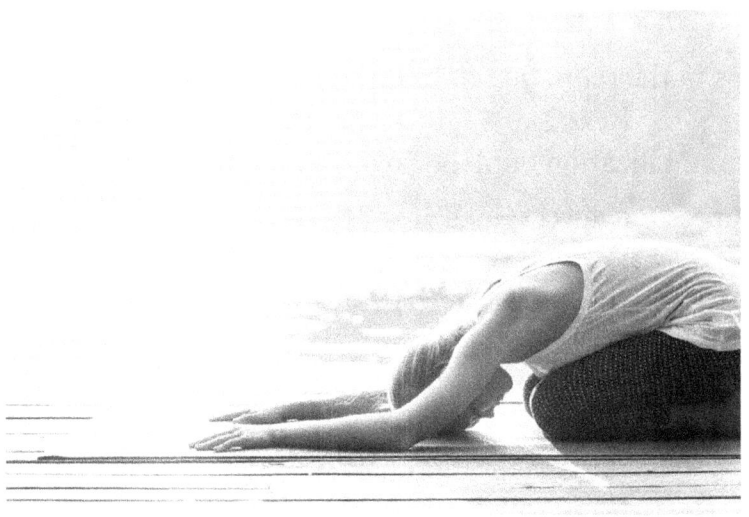

Over the years there have been approximately two hundred documented medical studies based on the Ashwagandha herb and these studies have concluded that some of the healing benefits of this herb include the following key points:

- Protection of the body's immune system; studies have shown that the use of this herb can result in the increase of white blood cell counts

- The treatment and resistance of the effects of stress, both external and internal

- Improvement of cognitive functions such as learning ability, memory and reaction time

- The reduction and treatment of anxiety and depression without the common side-effect of drowsiness that most chemical based treatments come with

- Aids in the reduction of brain cell degeneration

- The stabilization of blood sugar levels and helps to suppress sugar cravings

- The lowering of cholesterol

- Possesses many anti-inflammatory benefits

- Possesses anti-malarial properties

- Boosts and enhances libido and fertility in both men and women

- Useful in the preventative measures taken against cancer

- Helps to fight insomnia

- Helps with the pain management of arthritic joints

- Has a positive effect on the endocrine, cardiac and central nervous systems

- Can help the body maintain healthy thyroid function

- Possesses anti-oxidant properties

Before we dive into more benefits and uses of ashvagandha, I would like to offer you a free gift:

Free Complimentary PDF eBook

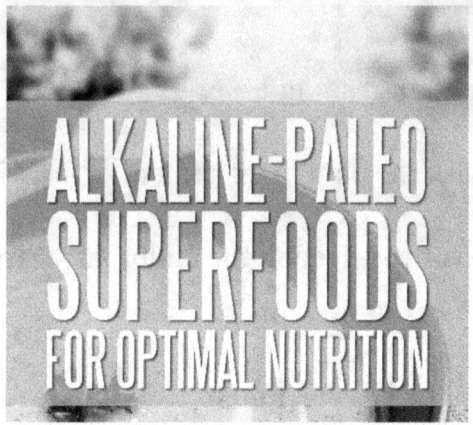

Download link:

www.YourWellnessBooks.com

Problems with your download?

Contact us: elenajamesbooks@gmail.com

We're here to help.

Chapter 1

The Uses and Benefits of Ashwagandha

This chapter will take a more in-depth look at the key points, uses and benefits of the Ashwagandha herb that were mentioned toward the end of the introduction. Each key point will be looked at separately in order to provide as much information regarding the uses and benefits of Ashwagandha with relation to the key point in question. The aim of this chapter is to show how this natural element of healing can be used to fight off, reduce and prevent many of the health risks and conditions that so many people are faced with in today's world.

Ashwagandha for the Immune System:

The modern world has evolved to a time in which we are all living fast-paced lives that involve many unavoidable stressors. These stressors are all around us and are linked to work, home life, school and university, money, health and wellness. Having a healthy immune system allows your body to protect itself from these stressors. Stress, both emotional and physical can put a serious strain on the body and therefore on the immune system, making it important for us to consistently do as much as we can to provide support to this system. As mentioned in the introduction, the practice and principles of Ayurveda include a balance of the mind and spirit together with a balance of the body.

One of the ways in which many of us cope with our daily stressors is through a consistent exercise routine, which is a very good way to combat stress. However for those of us who take our exercise and physical activities to levels that reach further than just everyday moderate exercise, it is important to remember that the fitter you are, the more physical strain your body is capable of undergoing, which will in turn result in your body being under a large amount of physical strain. Physical strain, even the healthy kind that comes in the form of exercise can put the immune system under pressure; therefore it is even more important for very active people and competing athletes to consistently boost their immune systems. Generally if you are choosing to live a healthier lifestyle by keeping active then your overall approach to your health would be one that is holistic and as natural as possible; furthermore, competitive athletes are known to prefer the avoidance of chemical based immune enhancers. This is where Ashwagandha will come in handy as it is a completely natural and safe immune system booster that will ensure that your body can fight off any infections that it may be at risk of contracting due to the physical strain it could be under during times of intense training.

Due to the fact that Ashwagandha has adaptogenic properties it is able to help with the modulation of the body's response to the internal and external stressors that can put the immune system under strain, leading to the risk of contracting everyday viruses and illnesses.

Ashwagandha has the ability to help improve and increase the white blood cell count which is another immune boosting property that it possesses. An optimum white blood cell count is necessary for a strong immune system because white blood cells help to fight infections by attacking viruses, bacteria and germs that invade the body; all things that we are consistently exposed to and cannot avoid as they are all around us in everyday life. The white blood cells could also be referred to as the body's sniffer dogs as they can detect hidden infections and undiagnosed medical conditions. Because the white blood cell count can fall and rise in and out of the healthy range without us knowing, it is important to consistently take measures, through our lifestyles, diets and supplementation to ensure that this particular blood cell count remains within an optimum range. The use of Ashwagandha will be very helpful in this case.

Ashwagandha for the treatment and resistance of the effects of stress, both external and internal as well as for insomnia:

External stressors tend to be the cause of internal stressors. Our daily lives are filled with so many of these stressors that in many cases they are completely unavoidable, but they are controllable.

Examples of external stressors would be our jobs, families, money, school, traffic jams, late busses, broken down trains, leaking pipes, the list could go on forever. Usually many of us can cope with all these external stressors, but sometimes their compound is just far too much to handle and can then begin to cause internal stressors.

Internal stressors are when the body begins reacting to the external stressors and this can lead to many health problems such as cardiac diseases, high blood pressure, diabetes, insomnia, depression and anxiety.

Ashwagandha is very useful in the treatment and prevention of stress and anxiety, helping you to better cope with the external stressors and therefore relieving and preventing the internal stressors that they cause. Ayurvedic healers acknowledge Ashwagandha for its calming effect on the central nervous system, since this herb is also a member of the nightshade family and it is revered within the practice for its ability to help the body adapt to stress and therefore help to prolong life. Within this ancient healing practice, Ashwagandha has been prescribed over centuries for its ability to ease anxiety, calm panic attacks, alleviate insomnia and reduce depression.

Medical research has revealed that Ashwagandha's relaxant properties are the result of it containing a group of alkaloids known as withanolides. Ashwagandha also contains alkaloids such as sitoindosides and saponins, as well as an assortment of essential minerals, all of which are believed to create a state of relaxation by working on the central nervous system as a depressant, resulting in sensations of relaxation and tranquility; both necessary states in order to achieve consistent and good quality sleepful nights.

Clinical studies in which subject suffering from severe anxiety proved that there was a far more effective decline in, and an increased ability to handle anxiety and stress among those subjects who were treated with Ashwagandha as opposed to those who were treated with psychotherapy alone.

Another clinical study surrounding subjects who were being treated for chronic stress proved that Ashwagandha treatment resulted in a substantial decrease of the stress hormone cortisol.

Ashwagandha for the improvement of cognitive functions such as learning ability, memory and reaction time, as well as the prevention of brain cell degeneration:

Overall sufficient cognitive function enables us to get through daily life far more efficiently then when we are in a constant state of brain fuzz. When our cognitive function is at an optimal level we are able to learn new things faster, remember things more efficiently, and have a much faster and more effective reaction time.

Part of the amazing journey of life is that we are constantly learning new things just by living in the world that surrounds us, however if we are consistently in a state of poor cognitive function we end up just existing rather than living and therefore miss so many of the things that are happening around us on a daily basis; these so-called things hold valuable lessons to our self growth. For example, simply observing the couple sitting next to at the coffee shop can teach you something new about people and their personalities, equipping you with stronger people skills. When you listen to a talk radio show or watch a talk show on television, you are being exposed to new and sometimes very relevant information about the world around you; however if your cognitive function is not firing on all, or most, of its cylinders then you will likely miss out on learning new facts and broadening your general knowledge.

It is well known that sufficient cognitive function is linked to good memory. A good memory is necessary in so many aspects of our daily lives, from remembering to put the food back in the fridge to remembering to lock the front door; a poor memory can lead to accidents and misfortune in so many ways. If your memory function is at an optimal level then you will be able to leave your grocery list at home, but still remember exactly what you need to buy purely because you wrote it down in the first place. Brain cell degeneration will cause you to have low and insufficient cognitive and memory function, which will also affect your learning ability.

In a clinical study surrounding the efficiency of Ashwagandha in promoting and increasing cognitive and memory function, while at the same time naturally reducing the possibility of brain cell degeneration; subjects were given doses of the Ashwagandha herb and then received a bout of psychometric testing. At the end of the two week trial all the subjects showed improvement in their reaction time, visual processing, memory function and overall brain health.

Ashwangadha for the stabilization of blood sugar levels and helping to suppress sugar cravings:

Unstable blood sugar levels and sugar cravings can be the result of many factors, including poor diet and lifestyle, as well as lifestyle related and hereditary diseases such as diabetes.

Studies have shown that the use of Ashwagandha aids in the metabolic process, therefore equipping the body with a stronger digestive system that will be able to efficiently and sufficiently break down all food substances in order to release the energy it is getting from them at a more optimal rate. When our energy levels drop due to hunger and insufficient nutrition, a drop in the levels of healthy sugar within our blood is a result. Blood sugar dips can cause headaches, nausea and in many cases irritability; all of which can lead to sugar cravings.

On the other hand, if our blood sugar rises too quickly, this will send our pancreas into overdrive, causing it to produce too much of the sugar regulating hormone, insulin. Consistent repetition of this state within the body can lead to type 2 diabetes, which is a chronic lifestyle related illness. Ashwagandha is known to help stabilize blood sugar levels keeping them from rising or dipping too fast or too high.

When our digestive systems and metabolisms are functioning at their peak then our bodies are able to reap all the nutritional benefits of the food that we are consuming. However it is important to note that even though Ashwagandha has been proven to aid and increase the metabolic and digestive process, it cannot erase the side-effects of a poor diet since a poor diet is a poor diet whichever way one looks at it. Ashwagandha would therefore be used as a supplement and a treatment in order to help get these systems within the body back on track and functioning at their peak.

Ashwagandha for the lowering of cholesterol, blood pressure and reduction of cardiac diseases:

Cholesterol is known as the silent killer as many of us don't know whether or not we are suffering from higher than normal or dangerous levels of bad cholesterol. High cholesterol can be caused by a number of factors that include hereditary disorders, bad lifestyle and dietary choices and chronic stress.

Ashwagandha has been known to effectively treat high cholesterol due to its ability to aid in the metabolic and digestive functions, helping the body to efficiently break down all the food that we eat. However, as with type 2 diabetes, if your high cholesterol is a result of a poor diet, Ashwagandha can only be used as a supplementation, preventative and treatment for your high cholesterol, and you would have to take all the factors that cause this state into consideration in order to effectively manage it.

Chronic stress can lead to high cholesterol due to the fact that it causes an increase in the stress hormone cortisol. Cortisol is known to affect a number of things within the body, including the healthy levels of cholesterol, therefore even if you are living a healthy life and following a nutritionally sound diet you could be at risk of high cholesterol if you are under chronic and server amounts of stress. This is where Ashwagandha's ability to help relieve stress has a double sided effect; by using this herb as a means to combat and manage your chronic stress situation, you are also in turn using it to help lower your cholesterol levels.

A combination of chronic stress and high cholesterol, as well as high blood pressure can lead to cardiac diseases by putting immense strain on the heart muscle and its regular function. Again there are a number of factors that can lead to high blood pressure and cardiac diseases, many of which include poor lifestyle and dietary choices as well. These too are conditions that can be managed without the use of chemical based drugs; through a lifestyle change that focuses on achieving sound health through diet, exercise, and stress management one can easily keep all these conditions under control. Ashwagandha can help in this situation on a number of levels due its stress relieving ability, as well as its digestive enhancing properties.

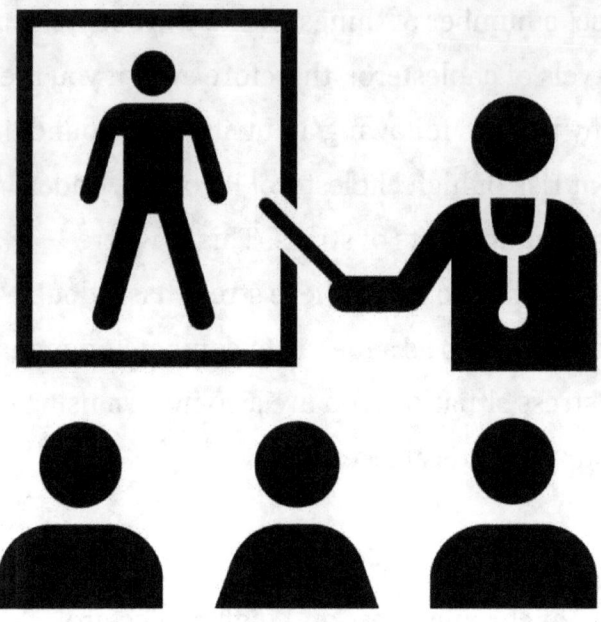

When one looks at high blood pressure on its own; there are many cases in our modern times where it is a result of our stressful lifestyles, here again it can be managed and prevented by the calming effects that come with the use of Ashwagandha.

Ashwagandha as an anti-inflammatory and for the pain management of arthritic joints and gout:

Inflammation within the body and its cellular makeup can lead to a number of health problems that include chronic cardiac diseases and a compromised immune system. Ashwagandha is known widely for its anti-inflammatory properties and therefore is a great addition to your daily routine in order to boost overall health and wellness in this aspect.

For those who suffer from arthritis and painful joints, Ashwagandha is a great remedy due to its anti-inflammatory properties. Arthritis is synonymous with an acid build up and inflammation within the joints and is usually caused by factors such as it being hereditary, a long-term side-effect of an injury, and the normal unavoidable aging process.

Gout is similar to arthritis in that is also caused by a high acidity within the joins and the body in general. This high acidity level can lead to pain and inflammation, which can be very effectively managed and remedied with the use of Ashwagandha.

Ashwagandha to boost and enhances libido and fertility in both men and women:

Ashwagandha is known for its potency when treating low libido and boosting the function of the fertility system in both men and women. When we have a healthy sex drive, we have a healthy reproductive system.

Fertility and the ability to conceive is very much affected by our stressful lives; there have been many cases where couples have been unable to conceive despite trying for a long time, and then suddenly once they relax about the situation the woman in the relationship is pregnant. Chronic stress can have a huge influence on fertility, and that's where Ashwagandha's stress reducing and stress treating properties play a role in the boosting of fertility. Also, when we are highly stressed and exhausted the last thing on our mind is intimacy, therefore our sex drive will naturally take a plunge.

Ashwagandha not only helps fertility and libido through its stress relieving properties, but also through its ability to promote healthy blood flow, therefore resulting in the treatment of impotence in men and the lack of lubrication in women. When our blood flow is pumping optimally around our system then our genitalia and reproductive systems are provided with enough healthy oxygen-rich blood, resulting in an increase in libido and fertility.

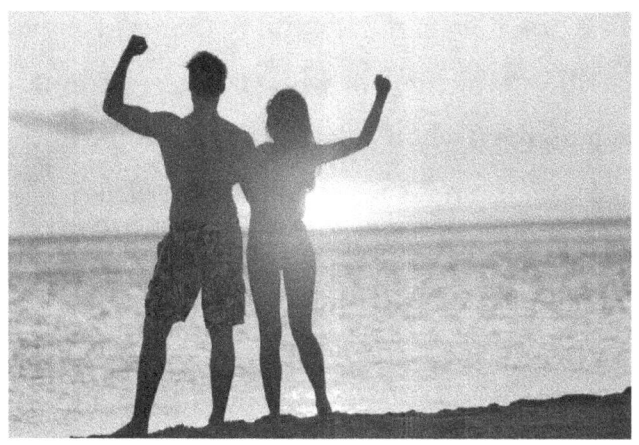

Ashwagandha for the prevention of cancer and as an anti-oxidant:

Due to its well-known high anti-oxidant properties and the fact that it is a known adaptogen, Ashwagandha has been shown, through numerous studies, to possess cancer fighting and cancer preventing properties.

Many of the cancer cases we hear about today are a result of the highly stressed lives we lead. Chronic stress leads to a compromised immune system and in so many cases it can, and does, lead to depression. There is an age old belief that unhappiness can lead to cancer, as the mind and soul is so strongly linked to the body.

Studies have shown that Ashwagandha's ability to increase the immune system's artillery which is our white blood cell count; it can be incredibly beneficial when used in conjunction with, and as part of, cancer treatment. These studies have also shown that Ashwagandha has the ability to promote the effects and efficiency of chemotherapy, resulting in a faster recovery time of certain types of cancers.

Further studies have shown that due to the alkaloids that make up the biochemical structure of Ashwagandha, it has the ability to reduce and prevent the growth of cancer tumors. It has also been discovered that this herb possesses cytotoxic properties against lung, colon, central nervous system and breast cancer lines.

Ashwagandha for the treatment of thyroid function and hormone rebalancing:

Due to its adaptogenic properties, Ashwagandha has been linked to, and in many cases proven to, aid in the optimum functioning of the thyroid and adrenal system, therefore rebalancing the body's hormonal system as well.

Ashwagandha has been known to help people with both hypo and hyper thyroid problems as it has been proven to treat and help both an over-active and an underactive thyroid gland. Ashwagandha was found to further benefit thyroid function due to its ability to greatly reduce lipid peroxidation through its ability to promote the destruction of free radicals that cause cell damage.

Due to its ability to fight and treat chronic stress, Ashwagandha has been found to be very supportive and useful in treating and strengthening the adrenal system, which is the system that is responsible for releasing the hormones cortisol and adrenaline; both of which are related to stressful situations. When you are under a chronic amount of physical, emotional and psychological stress your adrenal glands can take strain causing a condition that is known as adrenal fatigue. Adrenal fatigue can have a negative effect on the other hormones in your body such as progesterone which can then affect your fertility and cause you to age faster.

Ashwagandha's stress relieving, sedative, and carminative properties help to treat this adrenal fatigue and therefore promoting the rebalancing of your body's hormonal system, leading to more energy, increased libido and fertility, a stronger immune system, lowered and regulated blood sugar, lowered and regulated blood pressure, lowered and regulated cholesterol, and overall sound health for body, mind and spirit.

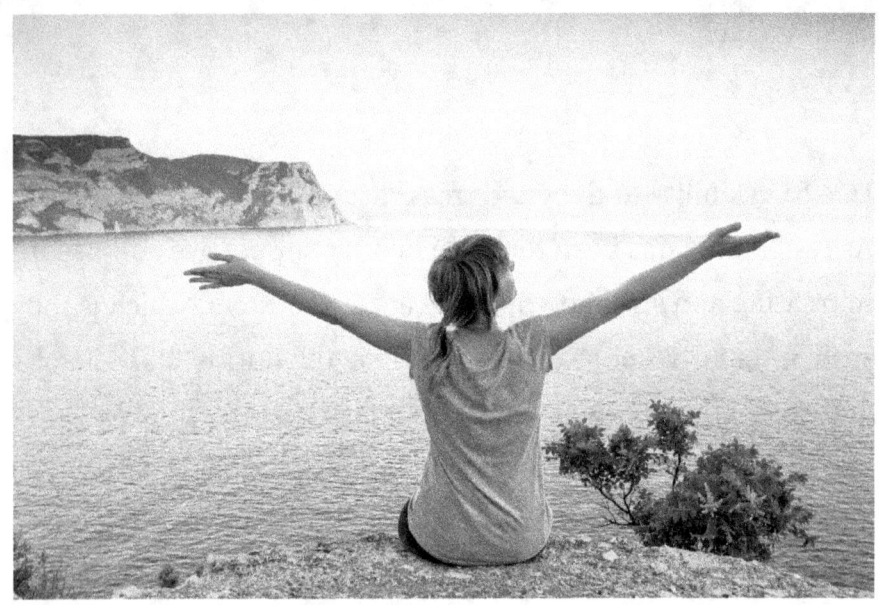

Chapter 2

Side-Effects and Precautions of using Ashwagandha

As with anything in this world, be it good or bad for the system, there are always going to be exceptions when it comes to the tolerance of certain medications, foods, and drinks. Although Ashwagandha possesses so many useful benefits to our overall health and the treatment of life's everyday upsets, there are also some side-effects that may occur while using this miracle herb, as well as some precautions that need to be taken into account. This chapter will look at these side-effects and precautions in order to make sure you are fully equipped with all the necessary knowledge around the use and application of Ashwagandha at all times.

Firstly it is good to note that the long term safety and side-effects of using Ashwagandha as an oral treatment are not completely known, however it is known that use of the herb as an oral medicinal compound in the short term has proven to be safe in general circumstances, but there is the possibility that overdose of the herb can lead to stomach upset, diarrhea and vomiting in some cases.

However it is advised to take certain precautions under the following circumstances:

- **When Pregnant or Breastfeeding:**

Due to the fact that there is not enough known about the use and side-effects of using Ashwagandha while breastfeeding, it is advised that it is completely avoided during this time. It is also suspected that there is a possibility that the use of Ashwagandha during pregnancy may lead to miscarriages so it is best to avoid the use of the herb completely during pregnancy.

- **In the case of Diabetes:**

Although Ashwagandha has many healing and useful properties when it comes to the prevention and treatment of diabetes, there are also cases when it has been known to interfere with prescribed Western medications for this particular lifestyle ailment. This interference has led to causing the blood sugar levels to drop too low, which can be very dangerous. It is always advised to consult with your physician before commencing treatment with Ashwagandha in order to ensure that you will not be putting yourself at any risk of the herb causing an interference with your existing treatment.

- **In the case of high or low blood pressure:**

Due to Ashwagandha's ability to help lower blood pressure, there is the risk that it may reduce blood pressure to a level that is too low in people who are already suffering from lower than normal blood pressure. Therefore you should take serious precautions when using Ashwagandha if you know that you have low blood pressure or if you are taking any medication for blood pressure in general. Again it is <u>highly advised that you consult with your physician</u> before commencing treatment with Ashwagandha to make sure that you are not putting yourself under any unnecessary risks.

- **In the case of stomach ulcers:**

There is a strong possibility that the use of Ashwagandha can cause irritation to the gastrointestinal tract. If you suffer from any kind of gastric disorders such as irritable bowels syndrome, crone's disease or a stomach ulcer it is advised that you either avoid the use of Ashwagandha completely or consult with your physician before commencing any treatment that involves the use of this herb.

- **In the case of Auto-Immune Diseases:**

If you suffer from or have been previously diagnosed with any of the auto-immune diseases such as multiple sclerosis, lupus, rheumatoid arthritis or any other disorder that is known to attack the immune system it is advised that you avoid the use of Ashwagandha as there is the strong possibility that it may increase the symptoms of these diseases. **Once again it is best to consult with your physician** if you are considering including Ashwangandha into your daily routine in order to reap its other benefits. There is an exception to every rule.

- **Ashwagandha and Surgery**

Ashwagandha has the ability to calm the central nervous system, which is a very good thing when using it as a treatment for stress and trauma, however in the event of surgery and post-surgery recovery there is the possibility that it may cause the central nervous system to slow down too much. There is also a strong concern that Ashwagandha may interfere with or cause a reaction with the anesthesia and other medications that are administered before, during and after surgical procedures. It is advised that you stop taking Ashwagandha at least two weeks before any scheduled surgical procedure **and of course you should consult with your physician**.

- **In the event of Thyroid Disorders:**

Even though Ashwagandha has many benefits when treating thyroid and hormonal imbalances and disorders, there is still the risk that it may increase thyroid hormone levels to a level that is not optimal. If you are using Ashwagandha as a treatment for thyroid or hormonal disorders it is advised that use it cautiously and **always consult with your physician** before commencing treatment. If you are taking thyroid or hormonal medications then it is advised that you avoid the use of Ashwagandha all together.

Chapter 3

Mouth-Watering Smoothie Recipes using Ashwagandha

The best, most efficient and easiest way to use and incorporate Ashwagandha into your daily life is by adding it in its powdered form to your smoothies. Ashwagandha powder is available at most health stores, pharmacies, and online. This chapter focuses on smoothie recipes that combine all the nutritional benefits of fruit, seeds, nuts, coconut; and in some cases super foods such as raw cocoa powder, Maca powder and Spirulina powder. All the recipes are completely vegan friendly so they are suitable for all walks of life.

As mentioned in the introduction; Ashwagandha is an herb that is used widely within the Ayurvedic practices of healing and balance of mind, body and soul, one of the key aspects of Ayurveda is sound nutrition and well balanced diet, these smoothies will help you achieve that. Many of the ingredients included in these recipes will not only help boost your immune system with their high nutritional content, but their high fibre content will also help you to achieve a healthy, well-working digestive system. Further benefits of the ingredients that have been included in these recipes include libido and fertility boosting properties.

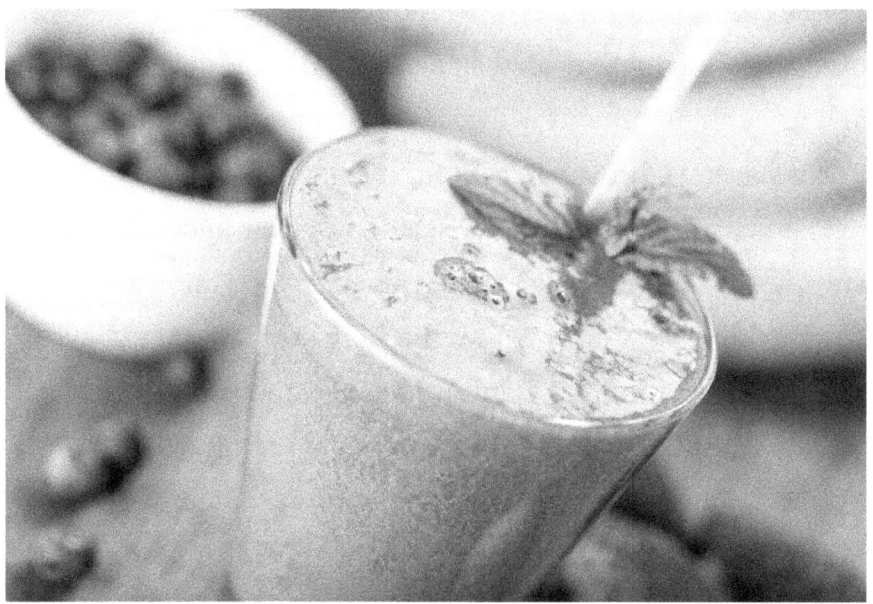

Libido Boosting Café Mocha Kick-Start Smoothie

Studies have shown that coffee reduces the odds of erectile dysfunction in men by increasing blood flow to the genitals, and its caffeine content will give you an energy boost. Raw Cocoa has been proven to contain the highest amount of anti-oxidants within one food source, and is a well-known natural anti-depressant. Maca is an ancient super food known to fight fatigue, increase energy, endurance and strength. Maca also stimulates the pituitary gland, which is responsible for secreting sex hormones. When combined with Raw Cocoa, Macca has synergistic effect. Cinnamon is used in Ayervedic healing because of its ability to promote healthy menstruation, and nourish the female reproductive system. Bananas are high in potassium and are known as a great natural energy source. The addition of Ashwagandha to this smoothie rounds off all the health benefits, making it not only good for boosting your libido and sex drive, but also adding a holistic approach to the ingredients.

Serves One:

Ingredients:

- 1 Cup (250ml) Almond milk
- ½ Cup (125ml) Organic filter coffee, preferably chilled
- 1 teaspoon (5ml) Tahini
- ¼ teaspoon (1.25ml) Vanilla Essence or extract
- ¼ teaspoon (1.25ml) Ground Cinnamon
- 1 teaspoon (5ml) Raw Cocoa Powder
- 1 teaspoon (5ml) Maca Powder
- 1 teaspoon (5ml) Ashwagandha Powder
- 1 medium sized banana
- 1 Tablespoon (15ml) chopped raw Hazelnuts

Instructions:

- Pour the almond milk and coffee into the jug of your blender.
- Add the Raw Cocoa, Ashwagandha and Maca Powders.
- Add the ground cinnamon, chopped Hazel nuts and Tahini.

- Add the vanilla essence or extract.

- Slice the banana into the jug.

- Blend until smooth.

- Since the almond milk does not require refrigeration, you can either drink this smoothie immediately, or pour it into a shaker to take away.

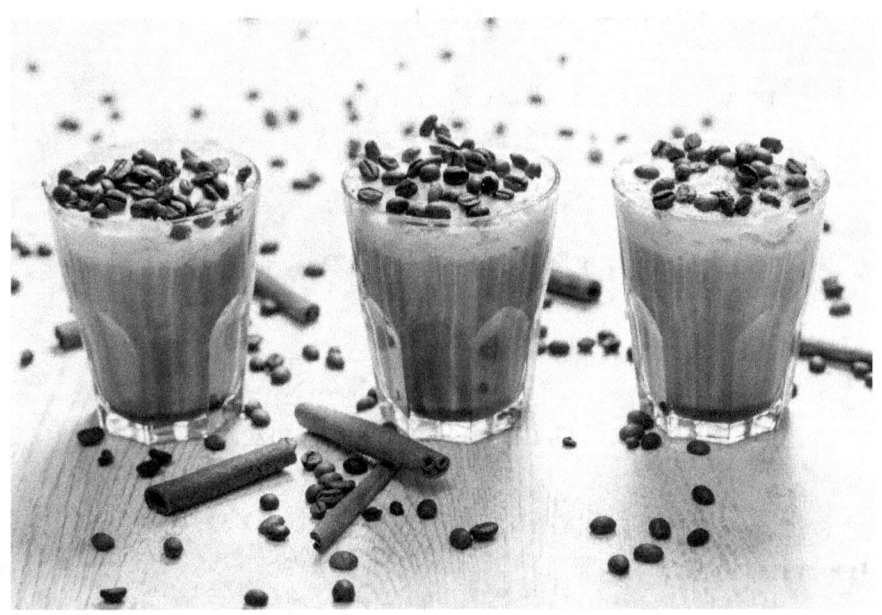

Apple, Date and Chia Smoothie

According to the healing principles of Ayervedic diets, apples are believed to work wonders for the sex drive, while dates help by combating fatigue, both fruits are high in the antioxidant vitamin C, so they add a cancer-fighting punch to the mix. Chia seeds are an ancient Mayan super food prized for their ability to provide sustainable energy. Chia seeds are also high in omega 3 fats, which are essential to a healthy female reproductive system and a strong immune system. Oat milk is high in calcium, which is essential for strong bone structure.

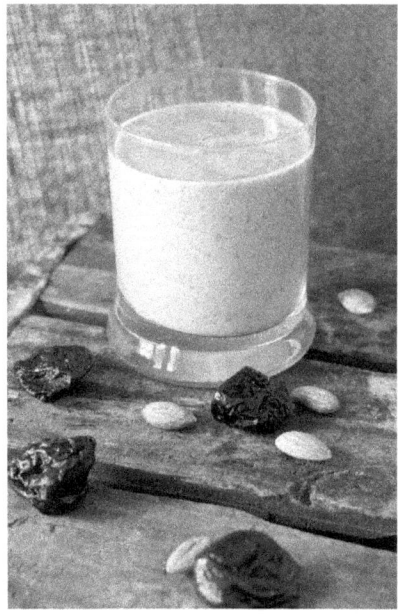

This smoothie uses a combination of oat and Chia seed milk, and requires a little preparation of ingredients prior to putting the actual smoothie together.

Serves One:

To make the Chia Seed Milk:

Ingredients:

- 2 Tablespoons (30ml) Chia Seeds
- 1 Tablespoon (25ml) Chopped raw almonds
- ½ teaspoon (2,5ml) vanilla essence
- ½ teaspoon (2,5ml) ground cinnamon
- 2 ½ Cups (750ml) water

Instructions:

- Mix the Chia Seeds, almonds and ground cinnamon together in a large jug.
- Add the water and vanilla essence.
- Set aside until the Chia Seeds have expanded to make a liquid with a milky consistency.

To make the smoothie:

Ingredients:

- 1 Cup (250ml) Oat Milk
- 1 Cup (250ml) Chia Seed Milk

- 1 Medium sized apple, cored and diced (peeling the apple is
- Up to you)
- 1 teaspoon (5ml) Ground Cinnamon
- 1 teaspoon (5ml) Ashwagandha powder
- 1 teaspoon (5ml) Tahini
- ¼ Cup (60ml) Chopped Dates

Instructions:

- Pour the oat and Chia Seed milks into the jug of your blender.
- Add the diced apple, chopped dates, Tahini, Ashwagandha powder and ground cinnamon
- Blend together until smooth.
- This smoothie will be best consumed immediately.

Coco-Pine Alkaline Ayurvedic Smoothie

Pineapple is a great source of vitamins C, B1 and B6; it is also high in manganese and folic acid, which is a good booster to the functioning of the reproductive and immune system. Coconut milk and desiccated coconut provide essential fats, as does the Tahini paste, these essential fats are known to help increase good cholesterol levels and lower the bad ones, and therefore they are incredibly useful and healthy to the cardiac system and functioning.

Serves One:

Ingredients:

- 1 Cup (250ml) Coconut Milk
- 1 Cup (250ml) Diced pineapple
- 1 Tablespoon (15ml) Desiccated coconut
- 1 Teaspoon (5ml) Tahini
- 1 Teaspoon (5ml) Freshly ground ginger root
- 1 Teaspoon (5ml) Ashwangandha powder

Instructions:

- Place the coconut milk and diced pineapple into the jug of a blender

- Add the desiccated coconut, Tahini, and ground ginger
- Add the Ashwangandha powder
- Blend until smooth

Chocolate Apple and Banana Secret Smoothie

This smoothie packs the energy boosting benefits of apple, which is a fruit known for its high pectin content making it a lower GI option and a great choice when looking to sustain your energy throughout the day. Apples are also high in anti-oxidants and essential minerals. Bananas are high in potassium and are also a great source of slow releasing energy and dietary fibre, adding to the energy boosting and sustaining properties and benefits of this recipe. The Raw cocoa not only adds a chocolaty taste, but also brings along all its powerful antioxidants, known as a super food, raw cocoa is believed to be the only food source to contain such a high level of anti-oxidants in one serving.

Serves One

Ingredients:

- One small banana

- One small apple, cored and diced (peeling is optional)

- 1 Cup (250ml) Almond milk

- 1 teaspoon (5ml) Ground Cinnamon

- 1 teaspoon (5ml) Maca Powder

- 1 teaspoon (5ml) Raw Cocoa Powder

- 1 teaspoon (5ml) Ashwagandha powder
- ¼ teaspoon (1.25ml) Vanilla essence
- 1 teaspoon (5ml) Natural almond butter

Instructions:
- Slice the banana into the jug of a blender.
- Add the diced apple
- Add the almond milk
- Add the Maca powder, Raw Cocoa and Ashwagandha powders
- Add the almond butter, ground cinnamon and vanilla
- Blend until smooth.

Minty Mango Anti Cancer Spirulina Smoothie

Among other nutrients, mangos give a good dose of vitamin E, which has been known to help improve sexual health. Spirulina is a super food made from a natural alga, and is very high in proteins, anti-oxidants, essential amino acids, omega 3s and is also very rich in vitamins and minerals. There is a lot of research that shows coconut milk to beneficial in the prevention of a number of cancers, particularly prostate and breast cancers as it is very alkaline forming in the body.

Serves One

Ingredients:

- 1 Cup (250ml) Coconut Milk
- 1 Cup (250ml) Diced Mango
- 1 Tablespoon (15ml) Chopped fresh mint leaves
- 1 teaspoon (5ml) Spirulina Powder
- 1 teaspoon (5ml) Ashwagandha powder

Instructions:

- Pour the Coconut Milk into the jug of a blender.
- Add the diced mango and fresh mint leaves

- Add the Spirulina and Ashwagandha powders

- Blend until smooth

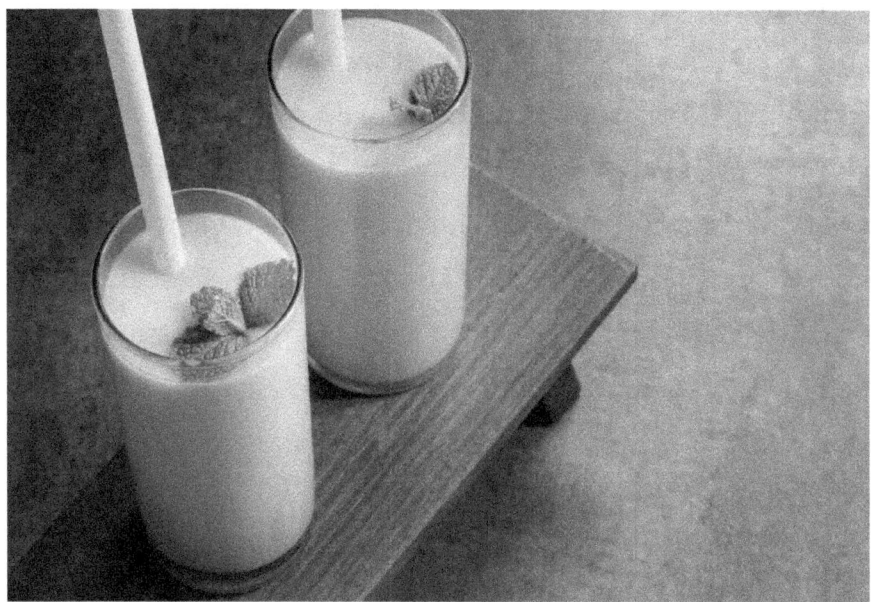

Strawberry Banana Oat Milk Smoothie

Strawberries are rich in folate, which is a B vitamin recommended for optimum pre-natal health, they are also high in anti-oxidants and offer many other nutritional benefits such as immune boosting qualities and a high vitamin C content. With the addition of the Shilajit powder, which is another herb that is used within Ayurvedic practices for the treatment of fertility and low libido, this smoothie is great for both men and women who are trying to conceive, especially considering that it also included all the fertility boosting benefits of the Ashwagandha powder. The energy provided by the banana will give you that extra boost and great dose of potassium.

Serves One

Ingredients:

- 1 Cup (250ml) Oat Milk
- 1 Cup (250ml) Chopped Strawberries
- 1 Medium Sized banana
- 1 teaspoon (5ml) Shilajit Powder
- 1 teaspoon (5ml) Ashwangandha Powder
- 1 Tablespoon (15ml) Chopped Raw Almonds

Instructions:

- Pour the Oat milk into the jug of a blender

- Add the chopped strawberries and slice the banana in to the jug as well

- Add the chopped almonds, Ashwangandha and Shilajit Powders

- Blend until smooth

Rice Pudding Smoothie

Rice milk is a great source of B vitamins and antioxidants. Blueberries also pack a good dose of vitamins, minerals and antioxidants and cancer fighting properties.

Serves one:

Ingredients:

- 1 Cup (250ml) Rice Milk
- 1 Cup (250ml) Blueberries
- 1 teaspoon (5ml) Ground Cinnamon
- 1 teaspoon (5ml) Ground Baking spice mix
- 1 teaspoon (5ml) Ashwangandha Powder
- 1 teaspoon (5ml) vanilla essence or extract
- 1 Tablespoon (15ml) Tahini

Instructions:

- Pour the rice milk into the jug of a blender
- Add the blueberries
- Add the ground cinnamon, spice mix, Ashwagandha Powder and vanilla. Add the Tahini and blend until smooth.

Super Antioxidant Anti Age Pomegranate Berry Smoothie

Goji Berries are not only super high in antioxidants, and cancer fighting properties. Acai berries originate from Brazil and are believed to increase overall energy and sex drive. Pomegranates are more widely known for their anti-aging properties, but have also been known to help improve skin health and are renowned for their ability to reduce the effects of aging within the cellular makeup of the body. Brazil nuts are thought to be one of the most concentrated sources of selenium, which has been linked to the improvement of testosterone levels as well as cognitive function. This recipe also contains Chia Seed milk, which will have to be made in advance.

Serves One:
To make the Chia Seed Milk:
Ingredients:
- 2 Tablespoons (30ml) Chia Seeds
- 1 Tablespoon (25ml) Chopped raw almonds
- ½ teaspoon (2,5ml) vanilla essences
- ½ teaspoon (2,5ml) ground cinnamon
- 2 ½ Cups (750ml) water

Instructions:

- Mix the Chia Seeds, almonds and ground cinnamon together in a large jug.
- Add the water and vanilla essence.

To Make the Smoothie:

Ingredients:

- 1 Cup (250ml) Chia Seed Milk
- 1 Cup (250ml) Almond Milk
- ¼ Cup (60ml) Goji Berries
- ¼ Cup (60ml) Acai Berries
- ¼ Cup (60ml) Pomegranate berries
- 1 medium sized banana
- 1 Tablespoon Chopped Raw Brazil Nuts
- 1 teaspoon (5ml) Maca powder
- 1 teaspoon (5ml) Ashwagandha Powder
- 1 teaspoon (5ml) Raw Cocoa Powder
- 1 teaspoon (5ml) Ground Cinnamon
- 1 teaspoon (5ml) vanilla essence

Instructions:

- Pour the Chia Seed milk, almond milk and vanilla essence into the jug of a blender.

- Add the all the berries and pomegranate

- Slice the banana into the jug

- Add the chopped Brazil nuts, cinnamon, Maca, Cocoa, and Ashwagandha powders

- Blend until smooth.

Coco-Pine and Cashew Nut Smoothie

Cashew nuts are high in heart healthy fats and protein. Pineapple is known for its high anti-oxidant and vitamin C levels. The coconut milk and cream bring along some extra heart healthy fats to the party as well as a tropical taste.

Serves One

Ingredients:

- 1 Cup (250ml) Coconut Milk
- ½ Cup (125ml) Coconut Cream
- 1 teaspoon (5ml) Vanilla essence or extract
- 1 Cup (250ml) Diced Pineapple
- 1 Tablespoon (15ml) Desiccated Coconut
- 2 Tablespoons (30ml) Chopped Raw Cashew nuts
- 1 teaspoon (5ml) Ground Cinnamon
- 1 teaspoon (5ml) Maca Powder
- 1 teaspoon (5ml) Ashwangandha Powder

Instructions:

- Pour the vanilla, coconut milk, and coconut cream into the jug of a blender

- Add the diced pineapple

- Add the desiccated coconut, raw Cashew nuts, ground cinnamon, Maca powder and Ashwangandha powders

- Blend until smooth

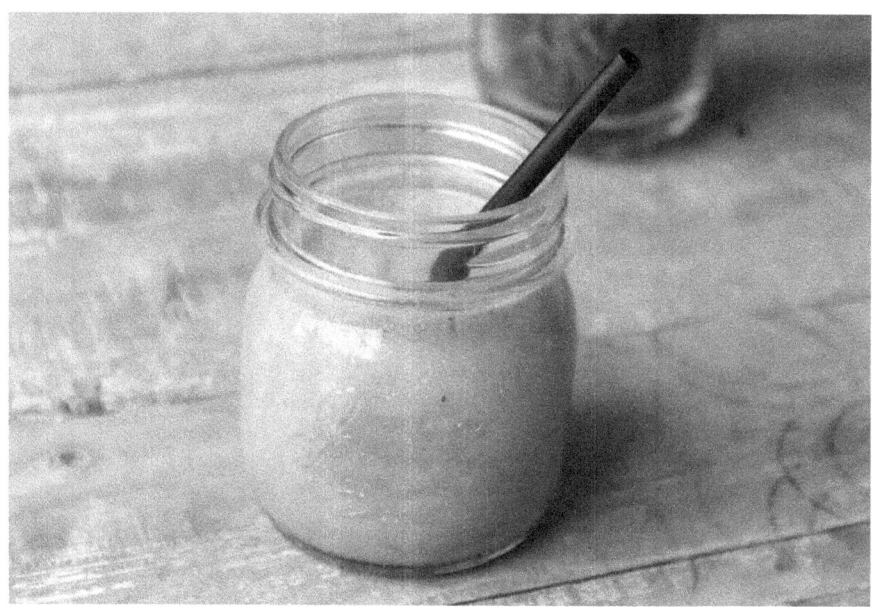

Green Apple and Pistachio Smoothie

This recipe uses green apples in particular purely for the colour aspect, don't be tempted to peel the apple for this one, as the rind will add extra fibre and colour to the end result. Certain studies have shown, that along with their cholesterol lowering abilities, pistachio nuts are also a great source of protein. Oat milk not only adds a creamy texture to this recipe, but it is also high in calcium and B vitamins.

Serves One:
Ingredients:
- 1 Cup (250ml) Oat Milk
- 1 large green apple cored and grated.
- 1 medium sized banana
- 2 Tablespoons (30ml) Chopped raw pistachio nuts
- 1 teaspoon (5ml) Spirulina powder
- 1 teaspoon (5ml) Ashwagandha Powder
- 1 teaspoon (5ml) Vanilla Essence

Instructions:

- Pour the Oat milk into the jug of a blender
- Add the grated apple and slice in the banana
- Add the chopped pistachios
- Add the Spirulina and Ashwagandha powders
- Add the vanilla
- Blend until smooth.

Carrot Cake Smoothie

The high fibre content of this smoothie will give you sustained energy. The carrots add a dose of vitamin A, and the Pecan nuts a high protein and zinc content which helps to balance hormones, by adding the Ashwagandha powder to this recipe this smoothie is a great option when you want to achieve an optimum hormonal balance within your body.

Serves One

Ingredients:

- 1 Cup (250ml) Rice Milk
- ½ Cup (125ml) Coconut Cream
- ½ Cup (125ml) grated carrot
- ½ Cup (125ml) chopped pineapple
- 2 Tablespoons (30ml) chopped raw Pecan nuts
- 1 teaspoon (5ml) ground cinnamon
- 1 teaspoon (5ml) baking spice mix
- 1 teaspoon (5ml) vanilla essence
- 1 Tablespoon (15ml) Raw oats
- 1 teaspoon (5ml) desiccated coconut

- 1 teaspoon (5ml) Ashwagandha powder

Instructions:

- Pour the rice milk, coconut cream and vanilla essence into the jug of a blender.

- Add the grated carrot and chopped pineapple

- Add the chopped pecan nuts, ground cinnamon and spices

- Add the desiccated coconut and raw oats

- Add the Ashwagandha powder and blend until smooth

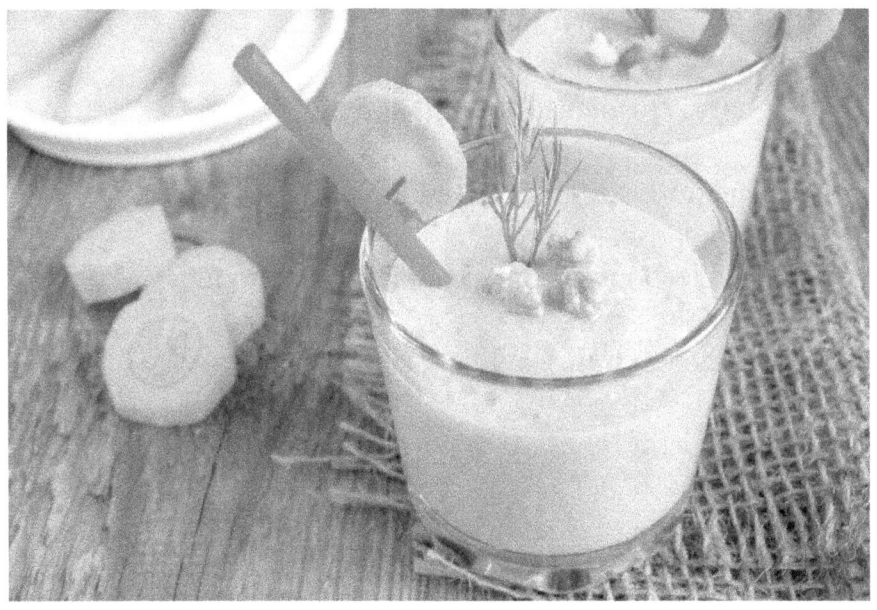

Peach Almond and Banana Smoothie

Almonds are high in omega 3 fats and contain the amino acid l-arginine, which helps transmit neurotransmitters to the brain, increasing sensations and cognitive function. Peaches are high in vitamin C, which is believed to boost libido in women, and their blood circulation boosting properties will help increase arousal. The addition of the Ashwagandha powder to this smoothie mix makes it a great source of libido boosting ingredients for any woman who is trying to increase her sex drive and conceive.

Serves one

Ingredients:

- 1 Cup (250ml) Almond Milk
- 1 Large fresh peach, pitted and diced
- 1 medium sized banana
- 2 Tablespoons (30ml) chopped raw almonds
- 1 teaspoon (5ml) vanilla essence
- 1 teaspoon (5ml) Maca powder
- 1 teaspoon (5ml) Ashwagandha powder
- 1 teaspoon (5ml) Raw cocoa powder

Instructions:

- Pour the almond milk into the jug of a blender
- Add the diced peach and slice the banana in
- Add the chopped almonds, Maca, Ashwagandha and Cocoa powders
- Add the vanilla
- Blend until smooth.

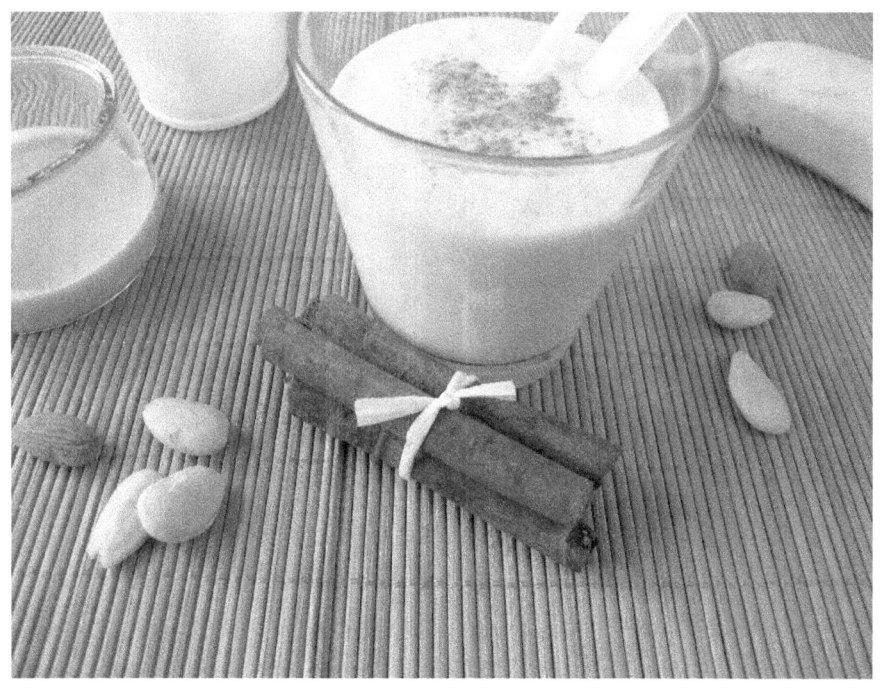

Potassium Punch Aztec Aphrodisiac Smoothie

Avocados were used by the Aztecs as sexual stimulants. This is a fruit that is high in folic acid and its healthy fat, potassium and vitamin B6 content boost hormone production as well as the strength of the immune system. Together with the nutritional benefits of the bananas, this smoothie combination is sure to give you long lasting energy. The high fibre content along with the lubricating benefits of the heart-healthy fats found in the avocado make this creamy smoothie a great stimulant for a healthy, well-working digestive system as well.

Serves One

Ingredients:

- 1 Cup (250ml) Rice Milk
- ½ Cup (125ml) Diced avocado
- 1 medium sized banana
- 1 Tablespoon (15ml) Tahini
- 1 teaspoon (5ml) Maca Powder
- 1 teaspoon (5ml) Ashwangandha Powder

Instructions:

- Pour the rice milk into the jug of a blender

- Add the diced avocado, and slice in the banana

- Add the Tahini, Maca and Ashwangandha powders

- Blend until smooth

Free Complimentary PDF eBook from Elena

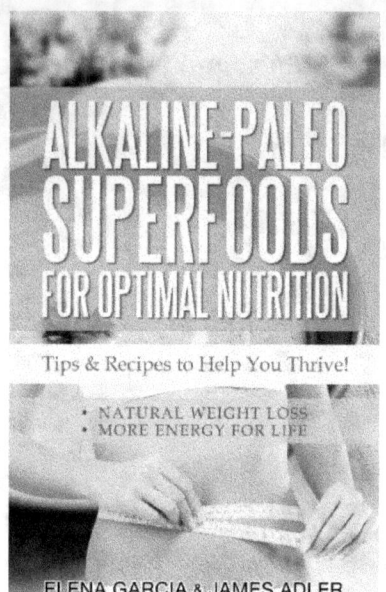

Download link:

www.YourWellnessBooks.com

Problems with your download?

Contact us: elenajamesbooks@gmail.com

In Conclusion

This book shows that there are many, many health and wellness benefits to the super herb known as Ashwagandha, further more the benefits of the Ayervedic practice and its healing methods are shown to be an efficient and natural way to achieve a holistic state of health for the mind, body and soul.

As mentioned in chapter 2, regarding the side-effects and precautions that need to be taken around commencing treatments that include the use of Ashwagandha, it is always advisable to consult with your physician before doing so as it is never a good idea to put your body and health at any risk.

We hope you enjoyed this book and are excited about taking care of your mind and body in a holistic way!

If you have a second, please rank this book on Amazon and post a short comment. Your opinion is very important to us and we would love to know your favorite recipe so that we can create more similar resources for you to enjoy.

Remember to take care of your lifestyle. Simply focus on one little change at a time and be good on yourself. Try to spend more time in nature. Disconnect from computers and technology as much as you can. Consider joining local yoga classes and embrace a positive mindset. Try to give yourself the luxury of sleep. We know that it may sound boring to many people- but going to bed earlier is one of the best natural cures you can imagine and it's free.

If you suffer from insomnia, the good news is that with Ashwagandha you can fight it very effectively without utilizing chemical medications and pills. For better results, we recommend you start using essential oils that are proven to help you relax: lavender, verbena, chamomile, sweet orange are great for that. Simply add 3-4 drops of your chosen essential oil to 1 tablespoon of coconut oil and add this mix to your bath, or use it for a self-massage after showering/bathing.

To learn more about simple healing rituals, including recipes and the essential oils, check out our other books (kindle & paperback editions available).

You will find them at: www.YourWellnessBooks.com

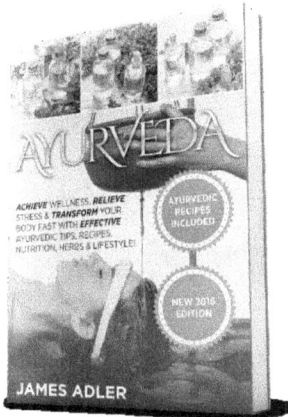 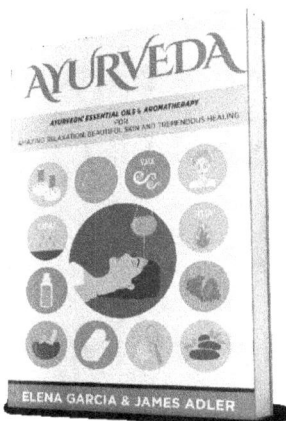

Welcome to Your Wellness Books family!

For more information and empowerment visit:

www.YourWellnessBooks.com

www.ingramcontent.com/pod-product-compliance
Lightning Source LLC
Chambersburg PA
CBHW071755080526
44588CB00013B/2248